COMPLETE GUIDE TO UNDERSTANDING ANGIOPLASTY

Comprehensive Handbook For Coronary Artery Procedures, Risks, Recovery, Advanced Techniques To Improve Heart Health And Longevity

KLEIN HOYLE

© [KLEIN HOYLE] [2024]

All rights reserved.

No part of this book may be reproduced, distributed, or transmitted in any form or by any means, including photocopying, recording, or other electronic or mechanical methods, without the publisher's prior written permission, with the exception of brief quotations in critical reviews and certain other noncommercial uses permitted by copyright law.

Disclaimer

The content in this book is based on the author's expertise and comprehension of the topic. The author has no affiliation or link with any corporation, business, or person. This book is meant to give general information and educational material only, and it should not be interpreted as professional medical advice. Always seek the advice of a skilled healthcare expert if you have any queries about medical issues or treatments. The author and publisher expressly disclaim any responsibility resulting directly or indirectly from the use or use of the information included in this book.

Table of Contents

CHAPTER 1 15
Introduction To Angioplasty 15
Definition And Purpose 15
Definition: 15
Historical Background 16
Overview Of Angioplasty Procedures 17
Pre-Procedure Preparation: 17
The Procedure: 18
Post-Procedure Care: 19
Importance Of Modern Medicine 19
Life-Saving Potential: 19
Widespread Use and Accessibility: 20
Quality of Life Improvement: 20
Economic Implications: 21

CHAPTER 2 23
Understanding The Cardiovascular System 23
Anatomy Of Heart And Blood Vessels 23
Function Of Arteries And Veins.....................24
Common Cardiovascular Diseases..................26
How Blockages Form 27

CHAPTER 3 29
When Do You Need An Angioplasty? 29
Symptoms Indicating Angioplasty 29
Diagnostic Tests (ECG, Stress Test, And Angiogram) 31
Risk Factors And Conditions That Require Angioplasty 32
Decision-Making Process 33

CHAPTER 4 37
Types Of Angioplasty..................................37
Balloon Angioplasty 37
How Is Balloon Angioplasty Performed? 37
1. Preparation: 37
3. Balloon Inflation: 38
4. Deflation and Removal: 38
Post-Operative Care 38
Stent Placement......................................39
How Stent Placement is Performed..............39
1. Simultaneous with Balloon Angioplasty: 39
3. Self-Expanding Stents:..........................40
Types of Stents.......................................40

Drug-Eluting Stents Versus Bare-Metal Stents...40
- Bare-metal Stents (BMS)..........................40
- Drug-eluting stents......................................41
- Choosing between BMS and DES 41

Alternative Techniques (Such As Atherectomy) .42
- Atherectomy..42
- How Atherectomy is performed....................42
- Benefits and Risks of Atherectomy 44
- After-Atherectomy Care 44

CHAPTER 5 47
Preparing For Angioplasty 47
Consultation Before The Procedure 47
Required Pre-Procedure Tests 48
Medication And Fasting Guidelines................49
Psychological Preparation 51

CHAPTER 6 53
The Angioplasty Procedure..........................53
Step-By-Step Guide To The Procedure.............53
- Preparation: 53
- Inserting the Catheter: 53
- Angiography: 54

- Balloon Inflation: 54
- Stent placement (if necessary): 54
- Assessment and Completion: 55
- Role Of The Medical Team 55
  - Interventional Cardiologist: 55
  - Anesthesiologist or Nurse Anaesthetist: 56
- Equipment And Technology Used 57
  - Catheters: 57
  - Balloon Catheter: 57
  - Stents: 57
  - Fluoroscopy Machine: 57
  - Monitoring Devices: 58
- Duration And Immediate Post-Procedure Care .. 58
- CHAPTER 7 61
- Postoperative Care and Recovery 61
- Hospital Recovery Process 61
- Monitoring And Follow-Up Appointments 63
- Medication And Lifestyle Changes 65
  - 1. Antiplatelet Agents: 65
  - 3. Blood Pressure Medications: 65
  - 4. Nitrates: 66

Identifying And Managing Complications 67
   1. Bleeding or Hematoma: 67
   2. Allergic response: 68
   3. Blood Clots: 68
   4. Restenosis: 69

CHAPTER 8 71
Risks and Complications of Angioplasty 71
Common Risks 71
   Bleeding 71
   Infection 72
Serious Complications 72
   Heart Attack 72
   Stroke 73
Long-Term Risks 74
   Restenosis 74
   Thrombosis 75
Preventive Measures 75

CHAPTER 9 77
Lifestyle Changes Following Angioplasty 77
The Importance Of Diet And Nutrition 77
Exercise And Physical Activity Guidelines 79

Stress Management Techniques 81
Regular Health Checkups 83
CHAPTER 10 87
Advances In Angioplasty And Future Directions 87
Innovations In Angioplasty Techniques 87
Development Of New Stents And Devices 88
The Role Of AI And Robotics 90
Conclusion 92
THE END 96

ABOUT THIS BOOK

The "Complete Guide to Understanding Angioplasty" is an invaluable resource for anybody wishing to expand their understanding of this crucial medical surgery. This book begins with a thorough introduction to angioplasty, including its purpose and historical evolution. It gives an overview of the different angioplasty techniques and emphasizes the importance of these treatments in contemporary medicine, stressing their role in saving lives and enhancing the quality of life for patients with cardiovascular disorders.

A thorough description of the cardiovascular system serves as a firm basis. This book methodically explains the architecture of the heart and blood vessels, including the functions of arteries and veins. It also dives into prevalent cardiovascular disorders and the processes that cause blockages, giving readers a thorough knowledge of the physiological issues that angioplasty seeks to overcome.

The explanation of when angioplasty is necessary is extremely informative. It discusses the symptoms that may signal the need for angioplasty, the diagnostic procedures used to validate these requirements (such as ECG, stress tests, and angiography), and the risk factors and circumstances that often need this intervention. The decision-making process is carefully examined, offering insights into how doctors evaluate if angioplasty is suitable for particular patients.

The guide differentiates between different forms of angioplasty, such as balloon angioplasty and stent insertion. It compares drug-eluting and bare-metal stents and provides alternative procedures like atherectomy. This section is quite useful for understanding the alternatives offered and their associated benefits and drawbacks.

Preparing for angioplasty is thoroughly discussed, including practical guidance on pre-procedure consultations, required testing, and medication and fasting instructions.

Psychological preparation is also addressed, emphasizing the emotional and mental components of going through a medical operation.

A step-by-step guide to the angioplasty technique is offered, emphasizing the role of the medical team, the equipment and technology employed, and what patients should anticipate in terms of time and immediate post-operation care. This openness helps to demystify the process, making it more accessible to patients and their families.

Post-procedure care and recuperation are crucial topics that are fully discussed. This book describes the hospital recovery process, the significance of monitoring and follow-up visits, and the drugs and lifestyle adjustments required for successful recovery. It also teaches how to identify and handle any difficulties.

The dangers and consequences related to angioplasty are openly explained. Common hazards include bleeding and infection, major consequences such as heart attack and stroke, and long-term problems such as restenosis and thrombosis. Preventive interventions are proposed to assist minimize these risks, providing patients with the information they need to take proactive actions in their treatment.

Lifestyle adjustments after angioplasty are emphasized as critical to long-term health. The significance of food and nutrition, exercise, stress management, and frequent health check-ups is emphasized, offering a comprehensive picture of post-angioplasty care.

Finally, This book looks forward, addressing advancements in angioplasty and possible future possibilities. Technique advancements, the creation of novel stents and devices, and the rising role of artificial intelligence and robots in angioplasty are discussed, providing a view into the future of cardiovascular treatment.

Overall, "Complete Guide to Understanding Angioplasty" is a comprehensive and important resource that covers all aspects of angioplasty, from comprehending the cardiovascular system and the need for treatment to the most recent breakthroughs in the field. This book is a valuable resource for patients, healthcare providers, and anybody interested in the changing landscape of cardiovascular therapy.

CHAPTER 1

Introduction To Angioplasty

Definition And Purpose

Definition: Angioplasty, commonly known as percutaneous transluminal coronary angioplasty (PTCA), is a minimally invasive technique for opening blocked or constricted coronary arteries. These arteries carry blood to the heart muscle, and blockages may result in angina (chest discomfort) or heart attacks. Angioplasty is the process of inserting and inflating a tiny balloon into an artery to enlarge it and enhance blood flow.

The main purpose of angioplasty is to restore enough blood flow to the heart, which relieves symptoms like chest discomfort and lowers the risk of heart attack. By expanding constricted arteries, angioplasty may improve a patient's quality of life and prevent the need for more invasive surgical treatments like coronary artery bypass grafting (CABG). Angioplasty is often done in combination with the insertion of a stent, a thin wire mesh tube that helps maintain the artery open in the long run.

Historical Background

Early Developments: While the idea of angioplasty extends back to the early twentieth century, substantial breakthroughs did not occur until the 1960s and 1970s. Dr. Andreas Gruentzig, a German cardiologist, pioneered the procedure's contemporary form by performing the first successful coronary angioplasty on a human patient in 1977. This innovation proved that coronary artery disease might be treated without requiring open-heart surgery.

Evolution & Milestones: Since Dr. Gruentzig's first treatment, angioplasty has seen countless adjustments and advances. In the 1980s, the invention of balloon catheters and guidewires improved the procedure's safety and effectiveness.

The introduction of stents in the 1990s was another key milestone. These little, extensible metal tubes offered a more permanent alternative for keeping arteries open. Drug-eluting stents, which release medicine to prevent re-narrowing of the arteries, have improved patients' long-term prognosis.

Overview Of Angioplasty Procedures

Pre-Procedure Preparation: Before an angioplasty, patients go through a series of measures, including diagnostic tests like coronary angiography, to assess the location and degree of their blockage. Patients are often advised to fast for several hours before the surgery and may need to discontinue certain medicines. A cardiologist who specializes in interventional procedures usually operates a catheterization lab.

The Procedure:

1. Catheter Insertion: The operation starts with inserting a catheter into a blood vessel, often in the groin, wrist, or arm. To numb the region, local anesthesia is administered, and the artery is accessed by a tiny incision.

2. Using real-time X-ray imaging (fluoroscopy), the catheter is carefully threaded into the blood arteries and directed to the location of the blockage in the coronary artery.

3. Balloon Inflation: Once the catheter is in place, a tiny balloon at its tip is inflated near the source of the obstruction. This balloon compresses the plaque against the arterial walls, enlarging it and restoring blood flow.

4. Stent Placement: A stent is typically put at the location of the obstruction. When the balloon catheter is inflated, the stent swells and stays in place to keep the artery open until the balloon is deflated and removed.

Post-Procedure Care: Following the angioplasty, patients are usually observed in a recovery area for a few hours. They may need to spend the night in the hospital for observation. Post-procedure treatment involves blood clot prevention drugs and follow-up consultations to assess the artery's status. Lifestyle adjustments, including eating a heart-healthy diet, stopping smoking, and getting regular physical exercise, are also critical for long-term success.

Importance Of Modern Medicine

Life-Saving Potential: Angioplasty has transformed the treatment of coronary artery disease by offering a less invasive alternative to open heart surgery. It has shown to be a life-saving operation, particularly in emergency cases such as heart attacks, when prompt treatment is critical.

By promptly restoring blood flow to the heart, angioplasty may reduce cardiac damage and increase survival chances.

Widespread Use and Accessibility: The technique is now widely available, with many hospitals and medical centers throughout the globe doing it. Advances in technology and technique have made angioplasty safer and more effective, with high success rates and low complication rates. This broad availability guarantees that more patients may get this life-saving medication.

Quality of Life Improvement: Aside from the immediate life-saving advantages, angioplasty dramatically improves patients' quality of life. Individuals may resume regular activities and have a higher quality of life by alleviating symptoms such as chest discomfort and shortness of breath. The method also lowers the need for more intrusive procedures, resulting in faster recovery periods and lower overall physical and mental stress for patients.

Economic Implications: Angioplasty is also economically advantageous. It lowers the long-term expenditures of treating severe coronary artery disease, which include hospitalizations and more costly procedures. By reducing serious cardiac events and facilitating faster recovery, angioplasty helps to create a more efficient healthcare system with reduced total expenditures.

CHAPTER 2

Understanding The Cardiovascular System

Anatomy Of Heart And Blood Vessels

The human heart is a muscular organ about the size of a fist that sits in the chest cavity between the lungs. It consists of four chambers: two atria on top and two ventricles on the bottom. The right atrium gets deoxygenated blood from the body via the superior and inferior vena cava. This blood is subsequently sent to the right ventricle, which circulates it to the lungs via the pulmonary arteries for oxygenation. Once oxygenated, blood returns to the left atrium via the pulmonary veins and is pushed into the left ventricle, where it travels to the rest of the body via the aorta.

Blood vessels are divided into three categories: arteries, veins, and capillaries. Arteries transport oxygen-rich blood out from the heart to the body's tissues, while veins return oxygen-depleted blood to the heart. Capillaries, the tiniest blood vessels, aid in the exchange of oxygen, carbon dioxide, nutrients, and waste materials between blood and tissues.

The coronary arteries are crucial because they deliver blood to the heart muscle itself. These arteries branch from the aorta and surround the heart. The proper performance and health of the coronary arteries are critical for the heart's functioning, since any blockages or abnormalities in these vessels may have a substantial impact on cardiac function.

Function Of Arteries And Veins

Arteries and veins serve diverse functions in the circulatory system. Arteries' strong, elastic walls are intended to withstand the enormous pressure of blood pushed from the heart. This arrangement allows them to keep blood pressure stable and move blood effectively throughout the body. The aorta, the biggest artery, divides into smaller arteries that connect to numerous organs and tissues. These arteries are further divided into arterioles and, finally, capillaries, which exchange nutrients and gases.

In contrast, veins have thinner walls and greater lumens than arteries. They work at a reduced pressure and include valves that prevent backflow, ensuring that blood flows in one direction—back to the heart. This venous system gathers deoxygenated blood from the capillaries and transports it via ever bigger veins until it reaches the superior and inferior vena cava, which drain into the right atrium of the heart.

The coordinated work of arteries and veins ensures that blood circulates continuously and efficiently, giving oxygen and nutrients to tissues while eliminating waste. Disruptions in this system may result in serious health problems, emphasizing the necessity of vascular function.

Common Cardiovascular Diseases

Cardiovascular diseases (CVDs) include a variety of illnesses affecting the heart and blood arteries. One of the most common CVDs is coronary artery disease (CAD), which develops when the coronary arteries constrict or block, limiting blood flow to the heart muscle. This disorder may cause angina (chest discomfort), heart attacks, and heart failure.

Another prevalent cardiovascular issue is hypertension (high blood pressure). It applies additional strain on the artery walls, possibly causing damage and raising the risk of heart attack, stroke, and renal disease. Atherosclerosis, which is defined by the accumulation of fatty deposits (plaques) inside the arteries, may cause these vessels to stiffen and narrow, increasing the risk of a heart attack or stroke.

Heart failure, a condition in which the heart is unable to properly pump blood, may be caused by a variety of underlying conditions, including coronary artery disease, hypertension, and cardiomyopathy. Arrhythmias, or irregular heartbeats, may affect the heart's rhythm and function, providing hazards that range from mild to fatal.

Other important cardiovascular disorders include valvular heart disease, in which one or more of the heart's valves fail to function effectively, and peripheral artery disease (PAD), which impairs blood flow to the extremities.

How Blockages Form

Atherosclerosis is a process that causes artery blockages, which are the leading cause of cardiovascular disease. This disorder starts with damage to the endothelium, which is the thin inner lining of the artery walls. High blood pressure, smoking, and high cholesterol levels are all risk factors for this kind of injury. When the endothelium is damaged, low-density lipoprotein (LDL) cholesterol may enter the arterial wall.

In reaction to this invasion, the body's immune system sends white blood cells known as macrophages to engulf the LDL cholesterol. Over time, these cells may transform into foam cells, which accumulate to produce fatty streaks. As this process continues, cholesterol, cellular debris, calcium, and fibrin (a clotting substance) accumulate on the arterial walls.

The plaque may continue to build, constricting the artery and reducing blood flow. If the plaque becomes unstable and ruptures, a blood clot may develop at the rupture site. A large clot may block blood flow, resulting in a heart attack if it happens in the coronary artery or a stroke if it occurs in an artery that supplies the brain.

Understanding how blockages arise emphasizes the need to maintain cardiovascular health with a healthy diet, frequent exercise, and quitting smoking.

CHAPTER 3

When Do You Need An Angioplasty?

Symptoms Indicating Angioplasty

Angioplasty is a treatment used to repair restricted or obstructed blood vessels, particularly the coronary arteries. It becomes essential when these arteries contract owing to atherosclerosis, a disease in which fatty deposits accumulate on arterial walls. Symptoms signaling the need for angioplasty are often caused by decreased blood flow to the heart muscle, which may lead to a variety of cardiac disorders.

One of the most prevalent symptoms is angina, which causes chest pain or discomfort. Angina symptoms include chest pressure, squeezing, fullness, or discomfort, as well as sensations in the arms, neck, jaw, or back. It usually happens during physical exertion or mental stress, when the heart's need for oxygen-rich blood rises but the restricted arteries can't give it.

In more severe circumstances, individuals may undergo a heart attack, also known as myocardial infarction. This happens when a coronary artery is fully stopped, preventing blood flow to a portion of the heart muscle. Heart attack symptoms include chest pain or discomfort that may extend to the arms, neck, jaw, back, or stomach, as well as shortness of breath, perspiration, nausea, and lightheadedness.

Furthermore, some people may not develop symptoms until the blockage is severe, resulting in a silent heart attack or sudden cardiac arrest. These instances highlight the necessity of prompt diagnostic testing and aggressive treatment in detecting and addressing possible blockages before they worsen.

Diagnostic Tests (ECG, Stress Test, And Angiogram)

Several diagnostic techniques analyze the heart's health and the amount of arterial blockages to decide whether or not angioplasty is necessary.

An electrocardiogram (ECG or EKG) is a noninvasive test that measures the electrical activity of the heart. It aids in detecting anomalies in cardiac rhythm, indicators of a past heart attack, or evidence of insufficient blood supply to the heart muscle.

A stress test, often known as a treadmill or activity test, assesses the heart's response to effort. This test involves the patient walking on a treadmill while their heart rate, blood pressure, and ECG are recorded. It may detect anomalies in heart function that may not be seen at rest, assisting in the diagnosis of coronary artery disease and determining the necessity for additional intervention.

Angiography, commonly known as coronary angiography, is an invasive technique used to see the coronary arteries. A contrast dye is injected into the arteries, and X-ray pictures are obtained to detect blockages or constriction. Angiography gives specific information regarding the location and degree of vascular disease, which helps guide treatment options like angioplasty.

Risk Factors And Conditions That Require Angioplasty

Several risk factors and underlying disorders increase the possibility of requiring an angioplasty to treat coronary artery disease.

High blood pressure (hypertension), high cholesterol levels (hyperlipidemia), and diabetes mellitus are all risk factors for atherosclerosis, which is the leading cause of constricted arteries. Individuals with these diseases are more likely to develop arterial blockages and may need angioplasty to restore normal blood flow to the heart.

Smoking, obesity, and a sedentary lifestyle all contribute to the development and progression of coronary artery disease. Smoking harms the blood arteries and hastens atherosclerosis, while obesity and physical inactivity raise the risk of hypertension, diabetes, and dyslipidemia. Managing these risk factors via lifestyle changes and pharmacological treatment may help avoid or postpone the need for angioplasty.

Other factors, such as a family history of heart disease, old age, and certain inflammatory illnesses, might predispose people to coronary artery disease and need angioplasty.

Decision-Making Process

The choice to have an angioplasty is based on several variables, including the severity of the symptoms, the findings of diagnostic testing, risk factors, and general health. A multidisciplinary team of cardiologists, interventional cardiologists, and cardiac surgeons assesses each patient to identify the best treatment option.

For individuals with stable angina or mild to moderate blockages, conservative treatment with drugs and lifestyle adjustments may be adequate to control symptoms and lower the risk of problems. However, if symptoms continue after adequate medicinal treatment, or if the blockages are significant and impair heart function, angioplasty may be indicated to restore blood flow and boost cardiac health.

In emergency conditions, such as a heart attack, angioplasty is often done right once to unblock the blocked artery and minimize damage to the heart tissue. In many circumstances, time is important, and early intervention may dramatically improve results and minimize the risk of complications.

The decision-making process entails comparing the possible advantages of angioplasty against the dangers of the surgery, taking into account the patient's age, general health, and preferences. Shared decision-making between the healthcare team and the patient ensures that treatment plans are personalized to the patient's specific requirements and objectives, resulting in improved results and quality of life.

CHAPTER 4

Types Of Angioplasty

Balloon Angioplasty

Balloon angioplasty, also known as percutaneous transluminal angioplasty (PTA), is a technique that opens up restricted or obstructed arteries, which are usually caused by atherosclerosis. This treatment includes inserting a tiny balloon, which is then inflated to expand the artery and enhance blood flow.

How Is Balloon Angioplasty Performed?

1. Preparation: The patient is often given a little sedative to assist them relax. Local anesthesia is used to numb the place where the catheter will be put, which is often the groin or wrist.

2. A tiny, flexible tube known as a catheter is placed via a small incision in the numbed region. The

catheter is carefully directed through the blood arteries to the location of the blockage using fluoroscopy, a sort of X-ray imaging.

3. Balloon Inflation: Once the catheter has reached the blocked artery, a smaller catheter with a deflated balloon at the tip is pushed through the first catheter to the source of the blockage. The balloon is then inflated, squeezing the plaque against the arterial walls while expanding the artery to improve blood flow.

4. Deflation and Removal: Once the artery has been adequately expanded, the balloon is deflated and withdrawn using the catheter. The insertion site is then sealed and bandaged.

Post-Operative Care

After balloon angioplasty, patients are frequently kept in the hospital for a few hours or overnight. They may need to lay flat to avoid bleeding at the catheter insertion site.

Blood thinners and antiplatelet medications are often recommended to prevent clot formation. Regular follow-up consultations are required to keep the artery open and check overall cardiovascular health.

Stent Placement

To assist in keeping the artery open after it has been expanded, stenting is sometimes used in conjunction with balloon angioplasty. A stent is a tiny mesh-like tube that supports the arterial walls.

How Stent Placement is Performed

1. Simultaneous with Balloon Angioplasty: If a stent is required during angioplasty, it is usually installed on the balloon catheter. When the balloon is inflated, the stent swells and presses against the arterial walls.

2. The balloon is subsequently deflated and removed, but the stent stays in place, serving as a scaffold to

keep the artery open. The arterial wall will eventually mend around the stent, further stabilizing it.

3. **Self-Expanding Stents:** Some stents are engineered to expand autonomously after they are withdrawn from the catheter, eliminating the need for balloon inflation.

Types of Stents

There are two main kinds of stents: bare-metal stents (BMS) and drug-eluting stents.

Drug-Eluting Stents Versus Bare-Metal Stents

Bare-metal Stents (BMS)

Bare-metal stents are basic metal mesh tubes that offer mechanical support for the artery after angioplasty. They are successful in preventing the artery from collapsing, but they increase the risk of restenosis (re-narrowing of the artery) because tissue may grow over the stent, causing it to narrow again.

Drug-eluting stents

Drug-eluting stents are coated with medicine that is gently infused into the artery, preventing scar tissue formation and lowering the risk of restenosis. The medications used in DES are usually anti-proliferative, which means they prevent cell growth.

Choosing between BMS and DES

- DES are preferable for people at high risk of restenosis since they minimize scar tissue development.

- BMS are cost-effective and accessible, making them a viable option for budget-conscious scenarios.

- Patient considerations, such as general health, ability to adhere to long-term antiplatelet medication, and particular medical disorders, might influence the decision between BMS and DES treatment.

Alternative Techniques (Such As Atherectomy)

In addition to balloon angioplasty and stent implantation, several procedures for treating restricted or obstructed arteries exist. One such method is atherectomy.

Atherectomy

Atherectomy is the removal of plaque from the arterial walls. This is especially advantageous when the plaque is hard or hardened, and balloon angioplasty alone may not be effective.

How Atherectomy is performed.

1. Preparation and Catheter Insertion: Similar to angioplasty, a catheter is introduced into the artery via a tiny incision.

2. Plaque Removal: There are a variety of atherectomy devices, including:

Directional Atherectomy: A spinning blade removes plaque.

Rotational Atherectomy involves a high-speed revolving burr that grinds plaque into microscopic particles.

Laser Atherectomy is a procedure that vaporizes plaque.

Orbital Atherectomy: A revolving diamond-coated crown removes plaque.

3. Plaque Extraction & Removal: The removed plaque is collected and retrieved from the body via a catheter. The artery is next checked to verify that it is suitably clean.

Benefits and Risks of Atherectomy

- Benefits: Atherectomy is useful in treating complicated lesions, such as hardened plaques and those in peripheral arteries.

- Risks: As with any invasive operation, there are risks such as arterial perforation, embolism (blockage caused by loosened plaque), and the need for subsequent procedures.

After-Atherectomy Care

Patients need monitoring after atherectomy, much as they do after angioplasty. They may need blood clot prevention drugs as well as frequent monitoring of their artery health. Long-term success requires lifestyle modifications as well as medical therapy for underlying problems including high cholesterol and hypertension.

Understanding the different forms of angioplasty and associated methods offers a complete picture of the choices for treating arterial blockages. Each technique has unique uses, advantages, and concerns, enabling healthcare practitioners to personalize therapy to their patients' distinct requirements.

CHAPTER 5

Preparing For Angioplasty

Consultation Before The Procedure

Before having an angioplasty, you should have a full consultation with your healthcare team. This session is intended to verify that you are both physically and psychologically prepared for the surgery. During this session, your doctor will go over the specifics of the angioplasty process, including the risks, advantages, and anticipated results. They will also check your medical history, current medicines, and any allergies you may have to verify that the operation is suitable for you.

Your doctor may also do a physical examination and request further tests to evaluate your general health as well as the state of your heart and blood vessels. To learn more about the blockages in your arteries, you may have an electrocardiogram (ECG), echocardiography, or cardiac catheterization.

Furthermore, the consultation allows you to ask questions and voice any concerns you have regarding the operation. It is important to communicate openly and honestly with your healthcare team to ensure that you completely understand what to anticipate during angioplasty and to address any worries or anxiety you may have.

Required Pre-Procedure Tests

Before having an angioplasty, many tests may be required to assess your heart health and discover any underlying issues that may have an impact on the procedure's success or recovery. These tests give essential information to your healthcare team, enabling them to personalize the treatment to your unique requirements while reducing the risks associated with angioplasty.

Coronary angiography, also known as cardiac catheterization, is a frequent diagnostic that includes injecting dye into your arteries and capturing X-ray pictures to see whether there are any blockages or narrowings. This test assists your doctor in determining the position and severity of the blockages, directing them during the angioplasty operation.

In addition, your doctor may prescribe blood tests to examine your cholesterol, blood sugar, and kidney function, as well as for symptoms of infection or inflammation. These tests assist uncover any underlying issues that may need to be treated before angioplasty and ensure that your general health is optimal for the treatment.

Medication And Fasting Guidelines

Your doctor will give you particular medication and fasting requirements to follow in the hours coming up to the angioplasty operation.

It is critical to follow these directions exactly to guarantee that the operation is safe and successful.

To lessen the risk of bleeding during angioplasty, you will usually be advised to cease taking certain medicines, such as blood thinners or antiplatelet tablets, many days in advance. However, you must contact your doctor before ceasing any prescriptions, since quickly terminating some drugs might have negative consequences for your health.

Your doctor may also urge you to fast for some time before angioplasty to ensure that your stomach is empty during the treatment. This often entails not eating or drinking anything for a certain number of hours before the planned operation time. Following fasting rules is critical for avoiding problems including nausea, vomiting, and aspiration during angioplasty.

Psychological Preparation

Preparing for an angioplasty requires both physical and psychological preparedness. It is common to feel scared before having a medical operation, but there are tactics you may take to control your emotions and gain confidence in the process.

One effective strategy is to educate yourself on the angioplasty technique and what to anticipate before, during, and after surgery. Understanding the stages involved and the reasoning behind them helps allay your anxieties and doubts, allowing you to make educated choices about your treatment.

Furthermore, relaxation methods such as deep breathing, meditation, or visualization might assist decrease tension and anxiety before angioplasty. Engaging in activities that promote calm and well-being, such as spending time with loved ones, listening to music, or pursuing hobbies, may also help you psychologically prepare for the treatment.

Furthermore, communicating openly with your healthcare team and voicing any worries or anxieties you may have may give comfort and support throughout the pre-procedure phase. Your doctor and other healthcare specialists are there to answer your questions, address your concerns, and make sure you are comfortable and prepared for angioplasty.

CHAPTER 6

The Angioplasty Procedure

Step-By-Step Guide To The Procedure

Preparation: Before the angioplasty treatment starts, you will go through several preliminary measures. This entails donning a hospital gown, having an IV line put in for medicines and fluids, and maybe getting sedation to help you relax during the process.

Inserting the Catheter: The initial step of angioplasty is to put a catheter into a blood artery, generally in your groin. Your doctor will use local anesthesia to numb the region before making a tiny incision. Then, a thin, flexible tube known as a catheter is delicately inserted into the blood arteries to reach the blockage.

Using fluoroscopy, a form of X-ray imaging, your doctor will guide the catheter through your blood arteries until it reaches the restricted or blocked artery in your heart.

Angiography: Once the catheter is in place, contrast dye is delivered into the coronary arteries. This dye highlights the blood arteries on X-ray pictures, enabling the doctor to determine the location and degree of any blockages.

Balloon Inflation: Once the blockage has been identified, a tiny balloon at the catheter's tip is inflated and positioned into the restricted artery. The pressure from the inflated balloon pushes the plaque against the artery's walls, enlarging it and restoring blood flow.

Stent placement (if necessary): During angioplasty, a stent may be inserted. A stent is a tiny metal mesh tube used to keep an artery open. It is put over a deflated balloon and placed at the source of the obstruction. When the balloon is inflated, the stent expands and locks in place, keeping the artery open.

Assessment and Completion: After the balloon is deflated and removed, your doctor will do another angiogram to ensure that blood flow has improved and the blockage has been effectively addressed. Once they are pleased with the findings, they remove the catheter and apply pressure to the insertion site to avoid bleeding.

Role Of The Medical Team

To guarantee that the angioplasty process is successful, a multidisciplinary team works collaboratively. Here's the breakdown of their roles:

Interventional Cardiologist: This is the main cardiologist who conducts the angioplasty. They are specifically educated in cardiology and have extensive experience utilizing catheters and other tools to treat coronary artery disease.

Nurses play an important role in aiding the interventional cardiologist during the operation.

They assist with patient preparation, monitoring vital signs, delivering medicines, and offering support and comfort.

Radiology technicians are responsible for operating imaging equipment, such as fluoroscopy devices, during procedures. They guarantee that the pictures are crisp and precise, allowing the interventional cardiologist to maneuver the catheter through the blood arteries.

Anesthesiologist or Nurse Anaesthetist: If sedation or anesthesia is necessary, an anesthesiologist or nurse anesthetist will administer and monitor the medication during the treatment. Their objective is to make the patient comfortable and pain-free during the angioplasty.

Other support workers, such as technicians and administrative professionals, may also be engaged in certain stages of the operation, such as equipment setup, paperwork, and patient transportation.

Equipment And Technology Used

Several types of equipment and technologies are required for conducting angioplasty.

Catheters: These thin, flexible tubes are introduced into the blood vessels to transfer instruments and drugs to the blockage.

Balloon Catheter: This specialized catheter contains a tiny balloon at its tip that may be inflated to compress the plaque and expand a restricted artery.

Stents: These tiny, metal mesh tubes are used to support the artery and keep it from collapsing during balloon angioplasty. They are often coated with medicine to lessen the likelihood of re-narrowing (restenosis).

Fluoroscopy Machine: This imaging device uses X-rays to provide real-time pictures of the blood arteries and catheters throughout the body.

It assists the interventional cardiologist in directing the catheter to the exact area of the obstruction.

Contrast dye is injected into blood arteries to make them visible on X-ray pictures during angiograms. It aids the medical team in locating obstructions and assessing blood flow.

Monitoring Devices: This category includes equipment that monitors the patient's vital indicators, such as heart rate, blood pressure, and oxygen levels, during the operation.

Duration And Immediate Post-Procedure Care

The time of the angioplasty treatment varies depending on the severity of the blockage and if other operations, such as stent implantation, are required. On average, the operation takes between 30 and 60 minutes.

Following the angioplasty, you will be brought to a recovery area and carefully monitored for any issues. You may need to lay flat for a few hours to stop bleeding from the insertion site, especially if no closure device was utilized.

Your medical team will offer instructions for post-procedure care, which may include:

• Limiting physical activity for a certain length of time.

• Taking prescription medicines, such as blood thinners and antiplatelet meds.

• Monitoring for symptoms of problems, including bleeding, edema, and chest discomfort.

• Consult with your doctor for additional examination and monitoring.

Most patients may return home the same day or after an overnight stay in the hospital. To guarantee the best possible result following angioplasty, you must follow your doctor's advice and attend all follow-up visits as scheduled.

CHAPTER 7

Postoperative Care and Recovery

Hospital Recovery Process

Following an angioplasty, you will normally spend some time in the hospital for healing and surveillance. The length of your stay will vary based on the intricacy of the treatment and your general health status. Throughout your hospital stay, you will be constantly followed to ensure that you are stable and recuperating well following the treatment.

Following the angioplasty, you will be brought to a recovery room where medical personnel will monitor your vital signs, including blood pressure, heart rate, and oxygen levels. To reduce bleeding and promote healing, you may also apply a tiny bandage or compression device to the catheter insertion site.

It is usual to feel groggy or drowsy in the first few hours after angioplasty because of the sedatives used during the surgery. You may also experience discomfort or minor pain around the catheter insertion site or where the balloon was inflated. The medical staff will provide pain treatment drugs to keep you comfortable.

As you begin to completely awaken from the anesthetic, you will be urged to slowly begin moving about. This helps avoid blood clots in your legs and improves circulation. However, you may be recommended to avoid vigorous activities for a while to enable your body to recover correctly.

During your hospital stay, you will be given post-procedure care instructions, such as how to care for the catheter insertion site, what activities to avoid, and any food restrictions that may apply. It is important to follow these recommendations precisely to reduce the risk of problems and encourage a quick recovery.

Before you are released from the hospital, your medical team will assess your status to verify that you are stable and ready to return home. They'll give you discharge instructions, including information about medicines, follow-up visits, and any issues to look out for. It is critical that you follow these directions and attend all planned follow-up visits to track your progress and address any issues as soon as possible.

Monitoring And Follow-Up Appointments

Following angioplasty, frequent monitoring and follow-up sessions are required to ensure that your heart health is adequately controlled and that any possible concerns are identified early on. Your healthcare practitioner will arrange follow-up consultations depending on your unique requirements and the details of your operation.

During these follow-up meetings, your healthcare practitioner will examine your healing progress, blood pressure, cholesterol levels, and general cardiovascular health. They may also conduct other tests, such as electrocardiograms (ECGs) or echocardiograms, to evaluate your heart's performance and identify any problems.

In addition to medical monitoring, follow-up sessions provide a chance to address any concerns or issues you may have regarding your recovery or continuing treatment. Your healthcare practitioner may advise you on medication management, lifestyle changes, and prevention methods for potential heart issues.

It is important to attend all planned follow-up visits and follow any suggestions made by your healthcare physician. These sessions are critical in ensuring that you get the necessary assistance and direction to keep your heart healthy and avoid issues.

If you suffer any symptoms or difficulties between planned sessions, such as chest discomfort, shortness of breath, or swelling at the catheter insertion site, call your healthcare professional right away. Early action is critical for resolving any difficulties and avoiding future health concerns.

Medication And Lifestyle Changes

Following angioplasty, your doctor may prescribe drugs to assist control your heart condition and lower the chance of future issues. These drugs may include:

1. Antiplatelet Agents: Aspirin and clopidogrel are often used to prevent blood clots from developing in the arteries, lowering the risk of a heart attack or stroke.

2. Statins and other cholesterol-lowering drugs may be administered to decrease LDL (bad) cholesterol levels and the risk of plaque development in the arteries.

3. Blood Pressure Medications: If you have high blood pressure, your doctor may give ACE inhibitors, beta-blockers, or calcium channel blockers to assist decrease your blood pressure and minimize the burden on your heart.

4. Nitrates: These drugs widen blood vessels, increase blood flow to the heart, and alleviate chest discomfort (angina).

In addition to drugs, lifestyle modifications are critical for preserving heart health and lowering the risk of future heart issues. Some essential lifestyle adjustments to consider are:

• Healthy Diet: Consuming fruits, vegetables, whole grains, lean meats, and healthy fats may decrease cholesterol, regulate blood pressure, and maintain a healthy weight.

• Regular physical exercise, such as walking, swimming, or cycling, strengthens the heart, improves circulation, and lowers the risk of heart disease.

Quitting smoking is a crucial step towards improving heart health. Smoking raises the risk of heart disease and might impede the healing process after angioplasty.

• Maintaining a healthy weight reduces stress on the heart and lowers the risk of obesity-related illnesses including diabetes and high blood pressure.

By adopting these drugs and lifestyle modifications into your daily routine, you may improve your heart health and lower your risk of future cardiovascular issues.

Identifying And Managing Complications

While angioplasty is typically a safe and successful operation, there are some possible risks. It is critical to be aware of these problems and understand how to identify and manage them.

Some potential consequences of angioplasty are:

1. Bleeding or Hematoma: Following angioplasty, you may have bleeding at the catheter insertion site or the development of a hematoma (a collection of blood beneath the skin). Monitor the insertion site for symptoms of bleeding or swelling, and get medical treatment if you detect anything unusual.

2. Allergic response: In rare situations, some persons may have an allergic response to the contrast dye used during angioplasty. An allergic response may include hives, itching, trouble breathing, or swelling of the face or throat. If you encounter any of these symptoms, you should seek medical assistance immediately.

3. Blood Clots: Blood clots may develop in arteries treated with angioplasty or at the catheter insertion site. These clots may partly or stop blood flow, resulting in significant problems including a heart attack or stroke. Follow your healthcare provider's antiplatelet prescription instructions carefully and report any blood clots symptoms, such as chest discomfort or shortness of breath, as soon as possible.

4. Restenosis: Following angioplasty, the treated artery may narrow again. This might be caused by scar tissue growth or plaque accumulation. If restenosis develops, other treatments such as repeat angioplasty or stent implantation may be required.

If you develop any symptoms or problems after angioplasty, you should seek immediate medical assistance. Early intervention may assist to avoid subsequent difficulties and increase the probability of a positive result. Your healthcare professional will collaborate with you to create a personalized treatment plan that will address any difficulties and improve your overall health and well-being.

CHAPTER 8

Risks and Complications of Angioplasty

Common Risks

Bleeding

Bleeding is a typical danger during angioplasty, especially at the insertion site where the catheter is put. During the surgery, a tiny incision is made to access the blood artery, which might result in bleeding. While moderate bleeding is normal and normally resolves on its own or with minimum intervention, severe bleeding may need medical treatment.

To reduce the risk of bleeding, your healthcare team will constantly examine the insertion site after the surgery and use pressure to stop any bleeding. You may also be recommended to refrain from engaging in activities that raise the risk of bleeding, such as heavy lifting, for some time after the surgery.

Infection

Infection is another possible complication of angioplasty, albeit it is uncommon. The catheter insertion site is the most likely source of infection. Although suitable sterilization measures are performed during the treatment to reduce this risk, infections may still arise, especially if the incision is not properly cared for afterward.

To limit the risk of infection, keep the insertion site clean and dry after the surgery. Your healthcare practitioner may give you information on how to care for the wound and what indications of infection to look for, such as increasing redness, swelling, or discharge.

Serious Complications

Heart Attack
While angioplasty is often used to enhance blood flow to the heart, there is a risk of heart attack during or after the treatment.

This may happen if the plaque accumulation in the coronary arteries is disrupted during the angioplasty procedure, resulting in a blockage or clot that prevents blood flow to the heart muscle.

To avoid a heart attack during an angioplasty, your healthcare team will carefully evaluate your risk factors and monitor your heart rhythm and vital signs during the treatment. In certain situations, further procedures, such as the implantation of a stent, may be used to assist in keeping the artery open and lower the risk of heart attack.

Stroke

Another major consequence of angioplasty is a stroke, which happens when blood flow to the brain is disturbed, either by a blockage or hemorrhage. The risk of a stroke during or after angioplasty is minimal, but it may occur if a blood clot develops during the treatment and travels to the brain, or if the neck arteries are injured during catheter placement.

To reduce the danger of a stroke, your healthcare team will carefully guide the catheter through the blood vessels while monitoring your neurological condition during the process. If you have a history of stroke or other risk factors, your doctor may recommend further precautions to lower your risk.

Long-Term Risks

Restenosis

Restenosis is a long-term danger related to angioplasty, in which the treated artery narrows again over time. This might happen as a result of scar tissue development or recurrent plaque accumulation in the artery. Restenosis usually happens within six months to a year after the treatment, although it may happen later as well.

To lessen the risk of restenosis, your doctor may prescribe antiplatelet medicines to prevent blood clots and statins to lower cholesterol levels. In certain circumstances, further treatments, such as repeat angioplasty or stent implantation, may be required to reopen the artery.

Thrombosis

Another long-term danger associated with angioplasty is thrombosis or blood clotting. Blood clots may develop inside the treated artery, especially around the site where a stent has been put, causing a blockage and restricting blood flow. Thrombosis might develop many weeks or even months following the surgery.

To lower the risk of thrombosis, your doctor may give antiplatelet drugs like aspirin or clopidogrel, which prevent blood clots from forming. It is critical that you take these drugs exactly as prescribed and that you see your doctor frequently to check for symptoms of clotting or other issues.

Preventive Measures

While angioplasty has dangers, patients may take preventative actions to reduce the consequences. A healthy lifestyle, which includes regular exercise, a balanced diet, and quitting smoking, may help lower the risk of cardiovascular disease and the need for angioplasty in the first place.

Furthermore, patients must carefully follow their healthcare provider's recommendations both before and after the treatment. This involves taking drugs as recommended, attending follow-up visits, and communicating openly with their healthcare staff.

Patients may undergo angioplasty with confidence if they understand the possible dangers and take proactive steps to avoid problems.

CHAPTER 9

Lifestyle Changes Following Angioplasty

The Importance Of Diet And Nutrition

Diet and nutrition are critical to recovery and long-term success after angioplasty. Following the treatment, it is critical to follow a heart-healthy diet to avoid future blockages and preserve general health. This entails concentrating on meals low in saturated fats, trans fats, cholesterol, and salt while prioritizing those high in nutrients such as fiber, vitamins, and minerals.

A heart-healthy diet often contains a variety of fruits and vegetables, whole grains, lean meats like fish and chicken, and healthy fats like nuts, seeds, and olive oil. These meals may help to decrease cholesterol, reduce inflammation, and enhance overall heart health. It is also critical to restrict the consumption of processed and fried meals, sugary beverages, and excessive quantities of red meat.

In addition to selecting the correct meals, portion management is essential. Eating smaller, more frequent meals throughout the day may help control blood sugar and avoid overeating. It's also vital to keep track of portion sizes and avoid super-sized meals, which may lead to weight gain and other health problems.

Along with nutrition, keeping hydrated is critical for heart health. Drinking enough water throughout the day may assist in removing toxins, controlling blood pressure, and enhancing general circulation. Aim to drink at least 8-10 glasses of water every day and restrict your use of sugary drinks and alcohol.

Overall, eating a heart-healthy diet and paying attention to nutrition may aid with angioplasty success and improve long-term cardiovascular health. By making wise food choices and adopting healthy eating habits, you may lower your risk of issues and live a better life.

Exercise And Physical Activity Guidelines

Regular exercise and physical activity are critical components of a healthy lifestyle, particularly after angioplasty. Regular physical exercise helps strengthen the heart, improve circulation, decrease blood pressure, and lessen the likelihood of subsequent blockages. To guarantee safety and efficacy, observe certain rules and precautions.

Before beginning any fitness program, talk with your healthcare physician to identify the best amount of activity for your specific requirements and medical history. Most persons who have had an angioplasty may safely participate in moderate-intensity activity such as brisk walking, swimming, cycling, or dancing.

Aim for at least 150 minutes of moderate-intensity aerobic activity each week, distributed over many days. In addition, perform strength training activities at least twice a week to help develop muscle and enhance overall fitness. Begin cautiously, then increase the intensity and length of your exercises as your strength and endurance develop.

It's also important to listen to your body and be aware of any warning signals or symptoms during exercise. If you feel chest discomfort, shortness of breath, dizziness, or excessive exhaustion, stop immediately and seek medical assistance as needed. Warm up before exercise and cool down afterward to avoid injury and boost healing.

In addition to planned exercise sessions, adding movement into your routine can help you remain active throughout the day. To improve your physical activity, use the stairs instead of the lift, park further away from your destination, or take brief walking breaks throughout the day.

Overall, frequent exercise and physical activity are critical for heart health and the effectiveness of angioplasty. By following these suggestions and remaining active, you may improve your general fitness, lower your risk of problems, and live a more fulfilling life.

Stress Management Techniques

Stress may have a substantial influence on heart health and general well-being, thus it is important to acquire appropriate stress management skills after angioplasty. Chronic stress may cause high blood pressure, inflammation, and other heart disease risk factors, so learning effective stress management techniques is critical for long-term heart health.

Deep breathing exercises are a very efficient stress management approach. Deep breathing may assist in soothing the nervous system, relieve stress, and promote relaxation. Regularly practice deep breathing techniques, inhaling slowly through your nose and exhaling through your mouth. Concentrate on breathing deeply into your belly rather than shallowly into your chest.

Meditation, gradual muscle relaxation, and guided visualization may all assist with stress management. Find a relaxation method that works for you and implement it into your daily routine to aid with stress reduction and general well-being.

Regular physical exercise is another strategy to reduce stress and boost mood. Exercise produces endorphins, which are natural mood enhancers that may help alleviate anxiety and despair. For stress relief, aim for at least 30 minutes of moderate-intensity exercise most days of the week.

It's also crucial to recognize and handle stressors in your life whenever feasible. This might include making lifestyle adjustments, establishing boundaries, or getting help from friends, family, or a mental health professional.

Remember that it is OK to seek assistance when necessary and that stress reduction measures may benefit both your physical and emotional health.

Integrating stress management practices into your daily routine may help lower the likelihood of problems and enhance long-term heart health after angioplasty. Prioritise self-care, develop healthy stress-management strategies and work towards a balanced and meaningful existence.

Regular Health Checkups

After angioplasty, it is critical to monitor your heart health and schedule frequent check-ups with your healthcare professional. Regular monitoring and follow-up treatment may help spot problems early on and prevent difficulties from developing.

During your check-ups, your healthcare practitioner will most likely do several tests and screenings to evaluate your heart health and track your progress.

This might involve blood tests to examine cholesterol levels and other indicators of heart health, as well as imaging tests like echocardiograms or stress tests to assess heart function.

In addition to physical checks and testing, your healthcare practitioner will review your lifestyle choices and provide advice on how to live a healthy life following angioplasty. This may include advice on food and nutrition, exercise and physical activity, stress management approaches, and medication management.

Communicate freely with your healthcare practitioner about any concerns or symptoms you may be having, and adhere to their recommendations for follow-up care and treatment. To obtain the greatest possible results, attend all planned visits and adhere to any recommended drugs or lifestyle adjustments.

In addition to frequent check-ups with your general care physician, you may need to visit additional specialists, such as a cardiologist or a cardiac rehabilitation team, for continuing treatment and support. These healthcare specialists can assist you in coordinating your treatment and providing extra resources and information to help you recover and maintain good heart health in the long run.

By being proactive about your health and scheduling frequent check-ups, you may help decrease the risk of problems and guarantee the long-term success of angioplasty. Take an active part in your healthcare, be knowledgeable about your situation, and collaborate with your healthcare team to attain and maintain good heart health.

CHAPTER 10

Advances In Angioplasty And Future Directions

Innovations In Angioplasty Techniques

In recent years, angioplasty procedures have advanced significantly, changing the way coronary artery disease is treated. One noteworthy advance is the creation of drug-coated balloons (DCBs). Unlike standard angioplasty balloons, DCBs deliver medicine directly into the artery wall to prevent restenosis, which is the re-narrowing of the artery after the treatment. This approach has shown encouraging results in preserving vessel patency for extended periods, minimizing the need for further treatments.

Another novel method is the use of biodegradable scaffolds. Unlike permanent stents, these scaffolds offer temporary support for the artery as it heals and is eventually absorbed by the body. This lowers the long-term risks associated with permanent implants, such as inflammation and late stent thrombosis. Clinical experiments have shown that bioresorbable scaffolds are effective in a variety of patient demographics, making them an attractive choice for future angioplasty treatments.

Furthermore, the use of intravascular imaging technologies like optical coherence tomography (OCT) and intravascular ultrasonography (IVUS) has improved the accuracy of angioplasty. These imaging modalities enable thorough visualization of the artery's inside, enabling for more precise stent insertion and evaluation of lesion features. This leads to better results and fewer procedural problems.

Development Of New Stents And Devices

Stents have been a staple of angioplasty for decades, and constant developments in their design have resulted in much better patient outcomes.

One significant advancement is the use of drug-eluting stents (DES). These stents are coated with drugs that suppress cell growth, reducing the creation of scar tissue, which may lead to restenosis. The most recent generation of DES features improved drug delivery systems and biocompatible coatings, hence increasing its safety and efficacy.

In addition to DES, specialized stents have been created for complicated instances such as bifurcation lesions and chronic complete occlusions (CTOs). Bifurcation stents are used to treat branching sites in arteries, keeping both the main channel and the side branch open. CTO stents, on the other hand, are designed to enter and sustain severely calcified or fully blocked arteries, opening up new therapy possibilities for patients who were previously deemed inoperable.

Bioresorbable and biodegradable polymer stents are examples of emerging stent technology. Bioresorbable stents, constructed from polymers such as polylactic acid, give temporary support to the artery before being progressively absorbed by the body, reducing the hazards associated with permanent metal stents. Fully biodegradable polymer stents provide comparable advantages while also breaking down into harmless byproducts during therapy, decreasing long-term issues.

The Role Of AI And Robotics

Artificial intelligence (AI) and robots are transforming the area of angioplasty by improving accuracy, efficiency, and patient outcomes. AI algorithms are being incorporated into diagnostic systems to help with the detection and evaluation of vascular abnormalities. These technologies can analyze imaging data with great precision, giving cardiologists crucial information for planning the surgery. For example, AI may assist in anticipating which patients are more likely to have issues, allowing for more targeted treatment techniques.

Another ground-breaking advancement is robotic-assisted angioplasty systems. These devices provide precise control of angioplasty instruments via a robotic interface, decreasing human error and boosting procedural accuracy. The operator can conduct complicated maneuvers with increased ease and stability, even in difficult anatomical situations. Furthermore, robotic systems limit radiation exposure for medical personnel by enabling them to operate from a distant console.

Furthermore, AI-powered platforms are employed to improve stent selection and placement. These systems analyze patient-specific data, such as vessel size and lesion characteristics, to suggest the best stent type and placement approach. This personalized strategy improves results while lowering the risk of restenosis or stent failure.

Conclusion

Understanding angioplasty, an important operation in the treatment of coronary artery disease is significant for both patients and healthcare practitioners. This thorough guide has clarified the numerous elements of angioplasty, including indications, procedures, advantages, dangers, and post-operation care, providing a well-rounded view of this life-saving treatment.

Angioplasty, also known as percutaneous coronary intervention (PCI), is the use of a balloon catheter to open restricted or obstructed coronary arteries, increasing blood flow to the heart muscle. The use of stents, and thin wire mesh tubes, has considerably increased the efficiency and longevity of this treatment, lowering the danger of arterial re-narrowing, also known as restenosis. Drug-eluting stents (DES), which release medicine to prevent scar tissue development, have improved patient outcomes by lowering restenosis rates.

The major reason for angioplasty is substantial coronary artery disease, which causes symptoms such as chest discomfort (angina), shortness of breath, or other signals of decreased blood flow to the heart. Angioplasty is especially important in the treatment of acute myocardial infarction (heart attack), because prompt restoration of blood flow may preserve heart muscle and increase survival rates.

While angioplasty has significant advantages, including fast symptom alleviation, increased quality of life, and decreased mortality in some settings, it is not without hazards. Although uncommon, complications might include bleeding at the catheter insertion site, artery damage, allergic responses to contrast dye, and, in certain circumstances, the necessity for emergency coronary artery bypass grafting (CABG). Long-term concerns include restenosis and stent thrombosis, emphasizing the significance of cautious patient selection and follow-up medical treatment.

Post-angioplasty treatment consists of lifestyle changes, medication adherence, and frequent follow-up. Patients are usually given antiplatelet medicines to prevent blood clots, cholesterol-lowering meds, and other medications to control risk factors including hypertension and diabetes. Lifestyle adjustments such as a heart-healthy diet, regular physical exercise, smoking cessation, and stress management are essential for sustaining the procedure's advantages and avoiding future cardiovascular problems.

Finally, angioplasty is a critical component in the therapy of coronary artery disease. The progression from basic balloon angioplasty to the present usage of sophisticated stents demonstrates substantial advances in cardiovascular therapy. Patients and healthcare professionals may collaborate to improve results and quality of life for people with coronary artery disease by understanding the procedure's complexities, hazards, and essential lifestyle changes. This handbook seeks to give the information required to negotiate the complexity of angioplasty, resulting in educated decision-making and comprehensive treatment.

THE END

www.ingramcontent.com/pod-product-compliance
Lightning Source LLC
Chambersburg PA
CBHW052332220526
45472CB00001B/386